How To Find Your Skin Type AndThe Perfect Products To Match

by
Jamelle Horsey

Table of Contents

INTRODUCTION

Finding the right skin care products can be difficult and confusing— especially if you're not sure what your skin type is to begin with. Skin types are typically determined by two factors: the condition of your skin and how easily it produces oils. In this guide, we'll explore the different kinds of skin, as well as how to tell which one you have and how to find products that match your uniqueneeds. One of the most important factors of beauty comes from healthy skin.

Healthy skin can be achieved if you take care of your skin and follow specific tips, depending on your skin type. Here are five secrets to achieving glowing skin that every woman needs to know!

Your skin is the largest organ of your body, which means that it's extremely important to take care of it, especially in the warmer months when you are sweating more and spending more time outside! Whether you have dry, oily, sensitive or combination skin, there are things you can do to help your skin stay healthy and beautiful. This guide to 5 secrets to glowing skin will show you how tokeep your skin soft and bright from head to toe. Knowing how to care for your skinis crucial, especially if you want it to look its best, but figuring out which products work best can be tricky. Knowing your skin type will help narrow down your options and you'll be able to quickly find the products that are worth using and those that aren't worth the space in your bathroom cabinet or on your bathroom countertop. Read on to learn more about the different types of skin and what you can do to achieve beautiful, healthy skin without breaking the bank!

Your skin type tells you everything you need to know about what productsto use, how often to apply them, and how likely they are to work well. The first step in achieving skin that's as healthy as it can be is taking the time to learn your skin type and which products would be best for it—but this can seem like an overwhelming task when all of the options available to you appear so different from one another. Use this guide on how to find your skin type and the perfect products to match to learn everything you need to know about your skin so that you can take control of its health and appearance!

Having the right products to care for your skin can make all the difference when it comes to preventing signs of aging and maintaining an overall youthful appearance. No matter what type of skin you have, though, it's important to choose products that are compatible with your unique complexion and needs. This guide to finding your skin type will help you learn how to find your skin type, figure out which products are best suited to treat your specific needs, and keep your skin looking young and healthy for years to come.

CHAPTER ONE

HOW TO IDENTIFY YOUR SKIN TYPE

What kind of skin do you have? Oh, that nagging query again. Though it may seem like a never-ending maze, finding the perfect skincare routine is the Holy Grail for many. Good news: it's not that difficult to figure out once you knowwhat to look for (and sort fact from fiction). Good thing you stumbled onto this page, because we can assist you with that. Here's a quick breakdown of the different skin types to

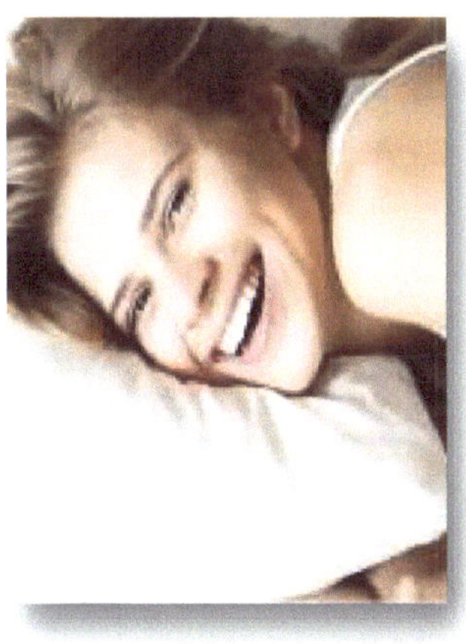

help you find your perfect match and start taking care of your skin.

Let's start off by putting some common misconceptions to rest. In reality, dry, oily, and mixed skin are the three distinct varieties of human skin. Acne and sensitivity are two more common skin problems that can affect anyone, but fortunately, they tend to clear up on their own. At any one time, anyone can have

any skin type and any skin problem. You may now learn more about your skin type and choose appropriate skincare products.

Is Your Skin Oily Or Dry?

The appearance of mixed skin, There is a good likelihood that those with combination skin will experience oiliness in the T-zone and dryness in the cheeks. Your nose's pores could also appear more pronounced than your cheeks'.

Reasons For Oily-Dry Skin

Simply said, having mixed skin indicates that you have more than one skin texture. Your nose, chin, and forehead pores tend to be overactive, which is the cause of the shine on those areas of your face, whereas the pores on your cheeks are less active and can cause a dry feeling. The sun, stress, and an insufficient amount of physical activity can all contribute to an increase in the severity of these indications. Some moisturizers also have the potential to clog pores.

How to treat skin that combines oily and dry elements

Even while it could appear as though you have the worst of both worlds, there is a simple technique to manage mixed skin that does not require you to spend a lot of time in the bathroom. What's the catch? You may easily customize your skincare routine to accommodate each of your skin's needs, or you can look for products that address a variety of issues at once. A micellar water like Simple Kind to Skin Micellar Cleansing Water is an excellent all-rounder that can easily remove make-up, oil, and debris without depleting skin of its natural moisture.

It is also important to be targeted in the way that you apply products. Why not choose more than one product based on the different issues you have? Instead of treating your entire face, you should only apply treatments to the specific areas of your face that require those items. Only your dry regions should be treated with a rich moisturizer; in order to prevent congestion on your oilier areas, you should tryusing a mask that provides a deep cleansing. Skin smarts? You got it.

These are the ingredients for different skin types:

For oily skin: Look for products containing alpha hydroxy acids (glycolic acid or salicylic acid), benzoyl peroxide, and hyaluronic acid. "These ingredients are effective at controlling excess sebum production while hyaluronic acid will produce hydration only in areas needed," Dr. Green says.

For dry skin: Look for products containing shea butter and lactic acid. "These ingredients provide hydration and mild exfoliation to keep dry skin looking radiant," Dr. Green says.

For sensitive skin: Look for products containing aloe vera, oatmeal, and shea butter. "They're good moisturizers and usually don't break anyone out," Dr. Greensays.

If you're not 100 percent sure what skin type you have. Once you understand your skin type, you can start selecting products from our website.

CHAPTER TWO

THERE ARE FIVE PRIMARY CATEGORIES OF SKIN: WHICHONE DO YOU HAVE?

"When it comes to identifying their skin type, the vast majority of people are deadincorrect." They are completely mistaken about whether they have dry skin or oilyskin, as well as whether or not they have sensitive skin. Because your skin type can shift over time and be influenced by factors such as climate, hormones, and diet, determining your real skin type can be a particularlychallenging endeavor. (There is also some disagreement as to whether or not "regular" skin and "sensitive" skin are really accurate descriptions of distinct skintypes.)

The following is some guidance from dermatologists on how to determine your personal skin type, as well as recommendations for skin care products, includingcleansers and moisturizers, for each of the skin types.

1. Oily skin

When a person has oily skin, their skin's natural process of producing oils might go into overdrive, which is especially likely if their pores are wider. This can cause the skin to become excessively greasy.

"The more active the oil glands are, the more they'll secrete when the pores are larger," This can result in a film of oil being left on your face for the duration of the day in addition to recurrent breakouts.

"You have oily skin if you notice that when you apply moisturizer, and pretty much anything else you apply, you break out," said Day. "If you observe this, youare more likely to have oily skin."

2. Dry skin

According to Day, having skin that is dull and lackluster is the most reliableindicator that you have dry skin.

The layer of dead skin cells that often covers dry skin is the primary reason of its lackluster appearance. If your skin is dehydrated, its surface will be rough and uneven, which will cause light to reflect in a variety of directions. On the other hand, if your skin is well hydrated, its surface will be smooth and uniformly reflectlight, which will cause it to appear more radiant.

Exposure to the sun, hot showers, and over-exfoliation with products containingsalicylic or glycolic acid are just a few of the many causes that can contribute todry skin.

According to Dr. Day, as we get older, our skin naturally becomes drier as a resultof changes in our hormones.

If you have a history of dry skin, the single most important thing you can do foryour complexion is to make sure it stays hydrated.

The simple act of hydrating the skin will cause it to appear younger, fuller, andmore radiant, according to Day.

3. Sensitive skin

"Sensitive skin is skin prone to irritation," Baumann explained.

Acne, rosacea, or contact dermatitis, which is a type of rash that is red, itchy, andcan occur in people with sensitive skin. She mentioned that people with sensitive skin were more likely to experience stinging or burning sensations.

She went on to say that those who have sensitive skin may have exaggerated reactions to particular components, and because of this, these individuals should steer clear of excessively harsh compounds in all of their cosmetic products, not just those pertaining to skin care. Isopropyl myristate, for instance, is a common component in hair conditioners, but persons who suffer from acne should steer clear of it.

People who have sensitive skin should steer clear of friction, extreme heat, and potential irritants such as alcohol or stress, according to Baumann, because these things have the potential to aggravate the condition.

According to Day, there is overlap between the categories of dry skin and sensitiveskin.

According to Day, "I consider dry skin to be sensitive as well." "Like, if you applyanything to it, it burns, it stings, and it goes red," she explained.

According to her, sensitive skin isn't necessarily a permanent skin type, but ratherone that can be caused if you overscrub, overexfoliate, or use products that are tooharsh. She says this because sensitive skin can be caused by doing any of these things.

According to Day, "most skin, provided that you use the

appropriate products, isnot as sensitive as you believe it is."

4. Combination skin

There is no one accepted definition of mixture skin, and some dermatologists, including Baumann, believe that it is not a genuine skin type in the same way thatoily and dry skin are.

According to Bauman, "skin type can alter with the seasons." "Having combination skin means that in the winter you are dry, and in the summer you are oily. This is considered to be an oily skin type, despite the fact that some individuals wrongly use the term to signify greasy in the T-zone.

Other physicians are of the opinion that mixed skin is a different skin type that can be identified by the variable amounts of oil that are produced on the face.

According to Day, "combination skin has a tendency to be oilier around the forehead and nose, where you have more oil glands, and drier on the cheeks." "The area surrounding the mouth is notorious for having a tendency to be both dry and oily, in addition to being more sensitive in general."

Day suggests applying a product that is formulated for oily skin on just the T-zoneof your face if you get the impression that this part of your face produces more oil than the rest of your face does.

She explained, "You can actually apply different products to the bridge of yournose and your forehead."

Alternating cleansers is another option, and you can do so based on whether your skin is feeling dry or oily at a particular time of the month or season.

This foamy cleanser from Restorsea is Day's go-to product for washing hercombination skin, and she highly recommends it.

5. Normal skin

As is the case with mixture skin, defining what constitutes normal skin can be difficult. Day makes the point that "normal" just refers to whatever is typical foryou.

She shared her thoughts on the matter with TODAY, saying, "I don't really think there is such a thing as 'normal skin.'"

You have your normal, which means that your normal will either be mixture, dry, or oily. I suppose that, if you want to construct a category, typical skin is skin that can withstand most things without overreacting.

Although Baumann acknowledges that there is no agreed-upon definition of "normal skin" in the medical field, one interpretation is that "normal skin" refers toskin that is both healthy and adequately moisturized.

"Normal skin produces sufficient sebum to moisturize the skin," she explained, "soin actuality, normal skin is oily skin with exactly the right amount of sebum production to keep skin healthy." **"Healthy skin"** might be a better descriptor, although even that doesn't refer to a real skin type.

Day has several items that she advises for those who don't have a tendency to have adverse reactions to the components of skin care products, despite the fact that normal skin might vary from person to person.

CHAPTER THREE

THE TRUTH ABOUT YOUR SKIN TYPE

There are a few popular skin types in the world, and each one has its ownset of benefits and drawbacks. If you're not sure which skin type you have, here's a breakdown of the most common ones:

➤ **Type 1**: This skin type is usually referred to as dry or sensitive skin. People with this skin type often struggle with acne and other skin problems.

➤ **Type 2**: People with this skin type are usually more resistant to skin problems. They may have more oily skin, but they're usually not as prone to acne.

➤ **Type 3**: This is the most common skin type. People with this skin type usually have normal skin that can handle a lot of wear and tear. They're usually not as prone to acne or other skin problems.

➢ **Type 4**: This is the rarest skin type. People with this skin type have the most oil production of any skin type. They also have the most sensitivity to the sun and wind.

There's a lot of information out there on skin types, but what does it all mean? Tostart with, your skin type is determined by the type of skin cells that make up your epidermis (outermost layer of skin).

CHAPTER FOUR

A GUIDE TO DEVELOPING A BASIC SKIN CARE TOINDIVIDUAL NEEDS

It would appear that the field of skin care is a complicated and ever-evolving one. However, the simplest skin care program could perhaps be the most effective foryou. It turns out that there are only three essential components to any routine.

"It's really intuitive," a professor of dermatology and cutaneous surgery at the University of Miami Miller School of Medicine told TODAY. "Cleansing is the first step. Second, you should apply some sort of moisturizer or hydrating solution. Third, shield yourself from the sun by applying sunscreen.

There are three main components of every skin care routine, andthey are:

➢ Cleanser

When getting ready in the morning or before bed, the first thing you should do is wash your face. Experts have also assured us that we might be less selective in our product selection.

Despite the fact that different skin types may have varied preferences, "you're never going to go wrong" with a simple, gentle cleanser, according to our product.Cleansers that don't contain any harsh chemicals (like salicylic acid) are ideal for those with dry or sensitive skin, and those that don't contain any fragrance are evenbetter. It's fine for most people's skin.

You may want to go back to a milder cleanser, I advised, if you begin incorporating other products into your routine that also include active components like these.Due to the potential for increased skin irritation or dryness, their combined usage is discouraged.

➢ Moisturizer

After washing and drying your face, I recommends using a

moisturizer to keep your skin moisturized and to strengthen its protective barrier.

The skin's protective function declines with age. Keeping your skin well hydrated and shielded from the elements is essential because "our skin doesn't regenerate or repair itself as much."

Even if you have oily skin, experts recommend moisturizing on a daily basis. However, you might find that a gel or water cream recipe is more to your liking due of its lightweight texture.

• Sun protection

The dermatologists recommend that everyone make applying sunscreen their last step in their morning skin care routine. Furthermore, you might be able to skip the

separate application of moisturizer and sunscreen altogether, as I suggested. People often use a cream or lotion as their morning sunscreen, which may be sufficient for your moisturizing needs.

Consistency is essential for success.

Following mastery of these three essential procedures, you can put in additional products or fine-tune your picks to address more particular skin conditions, such as hyperpigmentation or fine wrinkles. However, maintaining a constant routine of those three actions is of paramount importance.

This means only committing to a routine you know you'll stick with and resisting the urge to add new steps until you've mastered the basics. "Ideally, you're creating a regimen that you can feel comfortable using daily so that you really have consistency, because that's how you're going to see the benefit.

Using too many products at once might cause skin irritation (particularly if you're using many products containing active chemicals), and if irritation does occur, it can be difficult to determine which one caused it.

Newcomers to skin care, I stressed, should be patient. "There simply aren't any quick remedies," she sadly remarked. If you're starting a new routine, you shouldgive it a good six to eight weeks before giving up and buying more stuff.

If your skin care routine isn't helping you get your desired results, or if your skin iseasily irritated or prone to breakouts, you may want to try something else.

CHAPTER FIVE

THE BEST WAY TO CARE FOR YOUR SKIN TYPE

As a woman, you know that taking care of your skin is important. But withso many products and options out there, it can be hard to know where to start.

Here are five secrets to getting glowing skin that every woman needs to know

➢ Always moisturize your skin - it's the one thing that will make a world of difference in how you look and feel! There are several different ways to do this depending on what type of skin you have: use an oil- based moisturizer for dry or mature skin; use lotion for normal or combination skin; use gel for oily or acne-prone skin. You should also change up the routine throughout the year based on your climate: in summer months, go for lighter weight moisturizers; in winter months, use heavier moisturizers to protect against harsh weather conditions.

➢ Give yourself at least 10 minutes of me time each day - it'll help not only keep stress levels down but will also reduce wrinkles over time!

➢ Be sure to always wash your face before bedtime - even if you wearmakeup.

➢ Always exfoliate about once a week.
➢ Make sure to drink plenty of water (you should aim for 8 glasses perday).

A good rule of thumb is that if you're thirsty, then drink some water because it means your body is dehydrated. The American Academy of Dermatology recommends drinking eight glasses of water per day for healthy skin. In addition to hydrating our bodies, we need hydration from within. We need antioxidant protection from fruits and vegetables high in vitamins C and E as well as beta carotene found in carrots, sweet potatoes, apricots, spinach, kale and bell peppers. One very common mistake women make is they don't eat enough omega-3 fatty acids which are essential for radiant skin cells. What we put into our bodies matters!

DO NOT SKIP {SPF} SUN PROTECTION FACTOR

1.   The sun is your skin's number one enemy. It's important to wear sunscreen every day, even if you're just going to be inside. UV rays can penetrate through windows and cause damage.

2.   Pick the right sunscreen for your skin type. If you have oily skin, look for a gel or lotion formula that won't clog your pores. If you have dry skin, choose a creamformula that will hydrate your skin.

3.   reapply sunscreen every two hours, or more often if you're sweating orswimming.

4.   Exfoliate your skin regularly to get rid of dead skin cells and reveal radiant skin underneath. Use products made specifically for your skin type to avoid irritation. Take care of your nails too! They are not only an accessory but an indicator of health. Nails should not be weak, brittle, rough or chipped. Try to apply a coat of clear nail polish every week to protect them from the elements and keep them looking shiny and healthy! 5. Drink plenty of water! Water helps your body detoxify by removing toxins from your system and it also aids in repairing damaged skin tissue. Drink at least 8 glasses per day for best results.

Check out this youtube link

https://youtube.com/shorts/NFP5o5n8EP8?feature=share